Pharmacy OTC

By Babir Malik

About the author

Babir studied pharmacy at the University of Bradford and graduated in 2007 (after previously studying Biomedical Sciences at the same university). He joined Weldricks Pharmacy as a summer student in 2005, undertook his pre-reg with them and has stayed with them ever since.

Babir is now the Weldricks Pre-reg and Pharmacy Student Lead and Weldricks Teacher Practitioner, at the University of Bradford. He is also the Green Light Campus Northern Pre-Reg Lead, PCPA National Pre-reg Lead, Charity Ambassador for Pharmacist Support, Associate Fellow at HEA, as well as a tutor on the Royal Pharmaceutical Society Pre-Registration Conferences.

Babir currently practices as a relief pharmacist for Weldricks. In June 2016, the pharmacy that he co-managed at the time was awarded the Chemist and Druggist Medicines Optimisation Award for their innovative Local Pharmaceutical Service Intervention Service. He is a Chemist and Druggist Clinical Advisory Board Member.

As a Teacher Practitioner, his role includes being the MPharm Calculations Lead. Furthermore, Babir undertook a 10-week secondment as a Clinical Commissioning Group Pharmacist in North Lincolnshire early in 2016. He is also an OnTrack question writer and reviewer and is on the Medicines, Ethics and Practice Advisory Group. He completed his Clinical Diploma in Community Pharmacy at the University of Keele.

He can be found quite often on Twitter @Babir1981

Preface

If you are working in community pharmacy, then the amount of Over The Counter (OTC) information that you need to know can be overwhelming. All the information in this book can be looked up in a reference source but the more you know, the less you need to look up.

This book should be used after you have read an OTC textbook or your lecture notes and before attempting OTC multiple choice questions. It is also a fun way of refreshing your knowledge as pharmacist or pharmacy technician and could be used as tool to aid revision for university assessments and the registration assessment. Pharmacy technicians and counter assistants can also use it to quiz their responsible pharmacists!

There is a rationale to all questions and the majority contain a weblink for you to access more information. All the information was correct at the time of publication (March 2021) but please do ensure that you refer to the summary of product characteristics or patient information leaflet if attempting these questions after this date.

This book is not endorsed by the Royal Pharmaceutical Society or General Pharmaceutical Council.

Babir Malik

Acknowledgements

I would like to thank Joanna Domzal-Jamroz, Kat
Thorne and Natalie Jones for their kind assistance.

Foreword

I have known Babir for several years now. A friend, colleague, mentor, and a go to person for advice and guidance to many across the profession. His long history of involvement in all levels of pharmacy can be seen by the huge variety of work that he is involved in, particularly supporting students, trainees, and early careers pharmacists.

Some of the most notable things about Babir is his passion to help others while wanting to make learning a fun and enjoyable experience. This has led him to share his wealth of knowledge, expertise, and experience across a series of pharmacy related books. The latest addition to his growing authorship is *Pharmacy OTC Quizzes.* This book helps break down things into simple, concise, and easy to understand facts. As the role of the pharmacist continues to grow and expand, the confidence and trust from members of the public will too. This book helps you prepare for real-life questions you may get in your daily practice and will provide you with the confidence and explanations to help answer them.

I hope this book become a useful reference point to help with your current understanding while helping to identify any knowledge gaps you may have to facilitate further study.

Finally, I would like to congratulate Babir on his fantastic work, which will ensure future generations of pharmacists have the latest, up-to-date and evidence-based advice to support their daily practice and patient care.

Ravi Sharma, Director of England, Royal Pharmaceutical Society

1. Maloff Protect is taken once daily:
   True or False?

2. The maximum duration that Maloff Protect can be supplied without prescription is 8 weeks:
   True or False?

3. The minimum weight to be eligible to purchase Maloff Protect is 40 kg:
   True or False?

4. Maloff Protect contains atovaquone and chloroquine:
   True or False?

5. Chloroquine is taken once daily:
   True or False?

6. The Paludrine/Avloclor travel pack contains atovaquone and chloroquine:
   True or False?

7. The Paludrine/Avloclor travel pack contains enough for an adult for a four-week holiday:
   True or False?

8. Insect repellents containing DEET 50% are recommended:
   True or False?

9. The strength of Viagra Connect is 100 mg:
   True or False?

10. Sumatriptan is licensed for ages 18-60:
    True or False?

11. Chloramphenicol eye ointment should be kept in the fridge:
    True or False?

12. The minimum age for orlistat is 16 years:
    True or False?

13. The maximum age for orlistat is 60:
    True or False?

14. Orlistat 120 mg capsules are available OTC:
    True or False?

15. Esomeprazole, omeprazole, and pantoprazole are all P meds:
    True or False?

16. Chlorphenamine is no longer recommended for cough and cold in under 6s:
    True or False?

17. Simple Linctus is licensed from 6 years of age:
    True or False?

18. Simple Paediatric Linctus is licensed from birth:
    True or False?

19. Oral decongestants should not be used for more than 7 days:
    True or False?

20. Ipratropium is available OTC in a combination nasal spray with xylometazoline:
    True or False?

21. Hydrocortisone 2.5 mg Muco-Adhesive Buccal Tablets are available OTC:
    True or False?

22. Decongestants can cause drowsiness:
    True or False?

23. Sodium chloride nasal drops are safe to use from birth:
    True or False?

24. Coloured sputum is very common and indicates the need for antibiotics:
    True or False?

25. A patient with a cough lasting over a week should be referred to their GP:
    True or False?

26. Pink frothy sputum can be seen in heart failure:
True or False?

27. The MHRA advises that Codeine Linctus should not be used in children under 12:
True or False?

28. Dextromethorphan is more potent than codeine and pholcodine:
True or False?

29. The active ingredient in Simple Linctus is glycerol:
True or False?

30. Diphenhydramine is an ingredient in cough mixtures:
True or False?

31. Guaifenesin is a cough suppressant:
True or False?

32. 90% of sore throats are due to a bacterial infection:
True or False?

33. Patients who take carbimazole and present with a sore throat should be referred immediately:
True or False?

34. Infectious mononucleosis is common in the elderly:
True or False?

35. Presence of cough is part of the CENTOR criteria:
True or False?

36. Flurbiprofen lozenges are licensed from 12 years:
True or False?

37. Beechams All-in-One Oral solution contains 19% v/v alcohol:
True or False?

38. Acrivastine is a sedating antihistamine:
True or False?

39. Cetirizine can be used in children over 2:
True or False?

40. Loratadine can be used in children under 2:
True or False?

41. Acrivastine can be used in children over 12:
True or False?

42. Chlorphenamine can be used from 1 year in children suffering from an allergy:
True or False?

43. There are five steroid nasal sprays available OTC:
True or False?

44. Beclometasone, budesonide, fluticasone, hydrocortisone, and triamcinolone nasal sprays are available OTC:
True or False?

45. OTC steroid nasal sprays are licensed from 16 years:
True or False?

46. Azelastine nasal spray is available OTC:
True or False?

47. You can sell a pack of 24 x 30 mg pseudoephedrine tablets:
True or False?

48. Otrivine Extra Dual Relief Nasal Spray is licensed from 12 years:
True or False?

49. Lidocaine throat sprays are licensed from 12 years:
True or False?

50. Eye drops containing naphazoline can be used from 12 years:
True or False?

51. There are no ocular antihistamines available OTC:
True or False?

52. Chloramphenicol can be used OTC from 1 year:
True or False?

53. Chloramphenicol ointment should only be applied at night when used with drops:
True or False?

54. Chloramphenicol drops can be used for up to 7 days:
True or False?

55. Sodium cromoglicate drops should only be used once daily:
True or False?

56. There is a risk of severe and fatal burns with steroid creams:
True or False?

57. Oral lidocaine-containing products are GSL:
True or False?

58. Some head lice products are combustible/flammable when used on hair:
True or False?

59. Miconazole oral gel is contraindicated in patients who are taking warfarin:
True or False?

60. Overdose of loperamide can lead to serious hepatic events:
True or False?

61. Co-codamol 8/500 mg tablets can be used by a 12-year-old if they do not have breathing problems:
True or False?

62. Co-codamol 8/500 mg tablets are licensed for sore throats:
True or False?

63. The maximum pack size for paracetamol/dihydrocodeine tablets is 24:
True or False?

64. Paramol tablets contain paracetamol 500 mg and dihydrocodeine 10 mg:
True or False?

65. There is no treatment available for mild Otitis Externa OTC:
True or False?

66. Migraine with aura is classed as a primary headache according to the International Headache Society:
True or False?

67. Migraines are more common in men than women:
True or False?

68. Cluster headaches are more common in men than women:
True or False?

69. The most common type of headache seen in community is tension-type headache:
True or False?

70. Headache with aura is more common than without aura:
True or False?

71. Subarachnoid haemorrhages are more common in black people compared to other ethnic groups:
True or False?

72. Migraleve Pink tablets contain 8/500 co-codamol:
    True or False?

73. Buccastem M should only be used for a maximum of three days:
    True or False?

74. Buccastem M should be swallowed whole with a full glass of water:
    True or False?

75. Sumatriptan 100 mg is available OTC:
    True or False?

76. The maximum number of sumatriptan tablets that can be taken each day is two:
    True or False?

77. Diphenhydramine and promethazine tablets can only be sold to patients aged 18 and over for insomnia:
    True or False?

78. Alkalinizing agents for cystitis should be taken for 3 days:
    True or False?

79. Thrush has a thin white discharge and a strong fishy odour:
    True or False?

80. Clotrimazole pessaries should be used in the morning:
True or False?

81. Fluconazole oral capsules are licensed for use in women only:
True or False?

82. Vaginal thrush products can only be sold to those aged 16-60:
True or False?

83. Treatment with orlistat may potentially impair the absorption of water-soluble vitamins.
True or False?

84. No more than three orlistat capsules should be taken in a 24-hour period:
True or False?

85. Buscopan Cramps are contraindicated in patients with myasthenia gravis:
True or False?

86. The maximum daily dose of tranexamic acid is 3 g:
True or False?

87. Tranexamic acid should be used for a maximum of 3 days:
True or False?

88. The initial dosage of tranexamic acid tablets is one tablet three times a day:
True or False?

89. Painless mouth ulcers must be referred:
True or False?

90. Minor aphthous ulcers normally resolve in 2-3 days:
True or False?

91. Choline salicylate gel can be used from 6 years:
True or False?

92. Hydrocortisone Mucoadhesive Buccal Tablets can be used for up to 5 days:
True or False?

93. Chlorhexidine mouthwash can cause tooth discolouration:
True or False?

94. Daktarin Sugar Free 2% Oral Gel can be used from 1 year:
True or False?

95. When using Daktarin Sugar Free 2% Oral Gel, the treatment should be continued for at least a week after the symptoms have disappeared:
True or False?

96. Magnesium antacids can cause constipation:
True or False?

97. Aluminium antacids can cause constipation:
True or False?

98. Ranitidine can be used from 12 years:
True or False?

99. Proton Pump Inhibitors can be used from 16 years:
True or False?

100. Oral rehydration salts should be made with 200 mL water:
True or False?

101. The maximum daily dose of loperamide is 16 mg daily:
True or False?

102. Loperamide can be used from 6 years:
True or False?

103. Pepto-Bismol can cause black stools:
True or False?

104.   Kaolin and morphine is the first line treatment for diarrhoea:
True or False?

105.   There are three classes of OTC laxatives:
True or False?

106.   Lactulose is an osmotic laxative:
True or False?

107.   Ispaghula husk is a stimulant laxative:
True or False?

108.   Bulk-forming laxatives can take up to 72 hours to start working:
True or False?

109.   Stimulant laxatives take between 6-12 hours to work:
True or False?

110.   Glycerol suppositories work within seconds:
True or False?

111.   The standard dose of senna for adults is 3 tablets at night:
True or False?

112.   Ispaghula husk should not be taken at night:
True or False?

113.   Lactulose is not safe in pregnancy:
True or False?

114.   Docusate sodium is an osmotic laxative:
True or False?

115.   Hyoscine butylbromide can be used from 6 years:
True or False?

116.   Alverine and mebeverine can both be used in those over 12:
True or False?

117.   Peru balsam is a protectant used in haemorrhoids preparations:
True or False?

118.   Budesonide is available as a GSL nasal spray.
True or False?

119.   Haemorrhoid products containing hydrocortisone should only be used for a maximum of 7 days:
True or False?

120.   The most common form of psoriasis is scalp psoriasis:
True or False?

121.   Erythema means localised damage to the skin due to scratching:
True or False?

122.   There are four non-sedating antihistamines available OTC.
True or False?

123.   Ketoconazole shampoo should be used twice a week initially for the treatment of dandruff:
True or False?

124.   Terbinafine is an imidazole:
True or False?

125.   Daktacort Hydrocortisone cream is licensed from 10 years:
True or False?

126.   There are six classes of antifungal medicines available:
True or False?

127.   Amorolfine is used daily for distal lateral subungal onychomycosis:
True or False?

128.   Amorolfine is licensed from 18 years:
True or False?

129.   Toenails take approximately 6 months to regrow:
True or False?

130.   Each pack of amorolfine provides one month's treatment:
True or False?

131.   Minoxidil should be applied to the scalp three times daily:
True or False?

132.   Minoxidil 5% is only licensed for men:
True or False?

133.   Minoxidil is licensed from 18 years to 65 years:
True or False?

134.   Warts and verrucae are caused by the varicella zoster virus:
True or False?

135.   Salicylic acid products for warts and verrucae should be used once daily:
True or False?

136. Glutaraldehyde should be used once daily:
True or False?

137. Permethrin cream should be used from the neck down for scabies in all adults:
True or False?

138. Permethrin cream is licensed for use from 2 years:
True or False?

139. Cold sores are caused by the herpes simplex virus:
True or False?

140. Aciclovir cream should be used four times daily for five days:
True or False?

141. Penciclovir cream is used eight times daily:
True or False?

142. Hydrocortisone cream can only be used from 10 years:
True or False?

143. A maximum of 30 g hydrocortisone cream can be sold at one time:
True or False?

144. Hydrocortisone cream is available to buy for use on ears:
True or False?

145. Clobetasol cream is available to buy:
True or False?

146. Clobetasone cream can be used from 10 years:
True or False?

147. There is a combination aspirin and paracetamol product available OTC:
True or False?

148. Solpadeine Plus and Solpadeine Max contain the same amount of codeine:
True or False?

149. Ibuprofen suspension is available in 100 mg/5 mL and 200 mg/5 mL
True or False?

150. Dimeticone 4% lotion can be used from 1 year:
True or False?

151. Everyone in the house should be treated at the same time for head lice:
True or False?

152.   Head lice treatments should be re-
applied after seven days:
True or False?

153.   Head lice are only associated with dirty
hair:
True or False?

154.   Children with head lice should be kept off
school:
True or False?

155.   Isopropyl myristate can be used from two
years:
True or False?

156.   Isopropyl myristate should be left on for
30 minutes:
True or False?

157.   Everyone in the house should be treated
at the same time for threadworm:
True or False?

158.   Mebendazole can be used from 6
months:
True or False?

159.   The mebendazole dose for adults and
        children is the same:
        True or False?

160.   Infacol is safe to use from birth for colic:
        True or False?

161.   Gripe water is safe to use from birth:
        True or False?

162.   Colief contains simeticone:
        True or False?

163.   Emollients should be used sparingly:
        True or False?

164.   A three-year-old should take 7.5 mL of
        paracetamol 120 mg/5 mL oral suspension:
        True or False?

165.   A four-year-old should take 7.5 mL of
        ibuprofen 100 mg/5 mL suspension:
        True or False?

166.   Chickenpox is caused by the herpes
        zoster virus:
        True or False?

167.   Molluscum contagiosum is a bacterial
        infection:
        True or False?

168.   First line treatment for non-bullous
        impetigo is Crystacide cream:
        True or False?

169.   Glandular fever is caused by the Epstein-
        Barr virus:
        True or False?

170.   Scarlet fever is a viral infection:
        True or False?

171.   Roseola infantum is a viral infection:
        True or False?

172.   Roseola infantum is also called sixth
        disease:
        True or False?

173.   A blanching rash can occur with
        meningitis:
        True or False?

174.   German measles is also known as
        rubella:
        True or False?

175.   Mumps is much more unpleasant if
        contracted as a child:
        True or False?

176. Measles has an incubation period of one to two days:
True or False?

177. Koplik's spots occur in Measles:
True or False?

178. Scarlet fever is also called slapped cheek disease:
True or False?

179. Erythema infectiosum is also known as fifth disease:
True or False?

180. Glandular fever is a notifiable disease:
True or False?

181. Glandular fever is also called the kissing disease:
True or False?

182. Mumps is the most contagious of the childhood diseases:
True or False?

183. Joy-Rides can be used from 4 years:
True or False?

184. Kwells Kids can be used from 5 years:
True or False?

185.   Hyoscine does not cross the blood-barrier:
True or False?

186.   A Hyoscine patch is available for motion sickness:
True or False?

187.   Kwells can be used from 10 years:
True or False?

188.   EllaOne contains levonorgestrel:
True or False?

189.   EllaOne can be used in any female of childbearing age:
True or False?

190.   Ellaone can be used for up to 120 hours post unprotected sexual intercourse:
True or False?

191.   Ulipristal does not pass into breast milk:
True or False?

192.   Levonorgestrel can be used up to seventy-two hours post unprotected sexual intercourse:
True or False?

193.   If a patient vomits within four hours of taking levonorgestrel or ulipristal, a further supply would be needed:
True or False?

194.   Levonorgestrel is more efficacious than ulipristal:
True or False?

195.   A maximum of two nicotine inhalation cartridges can be used in 24 hours:
True or False?

196.   The maximum daily limit of nicotine nasal spray is 64 sprays:
True or False?

197.   Nicotine patches should be changed every seventy-two hours:
True or False?

198.   Crotamiton can be used from three years:
True or False?

199.   Large packs of stimulant laxatives are available GSL:
True or False?

200.   Children under 18 years must see a doctor if they require stimulant laxatives.
True or False?

Answers

1.   Maloff Protect is taken once daily:
Answer: True
Reference:
https://www.medicines.org.uk/emc/product/660

2.   The maximum duration that Maloff Protect can be supplied without prescription is 8 weeks:
Answer: False
Rationale: It can be supplied for 12 weeks.

3.   The minimum weight to be eligible to purchase Maloff Protect is 40 kg:
Answer: True

4.   Maloff Protect contains atovaquone and chloroquine:
Answer: False
Rationale: It contains atovaquone 250 mg and proguanil 100 mg

5.   Chloroquine is taken once daily:
Answer: False
Rationale: It is taken once weekly.
Reference:
https://www.medicines.org.uk/emc/product/5490/smpc

6.   The Paludrine/Avloclor travel pack contains atovaquone and chloroquine:

Answer: False

Rationale: It contains proguanil and chloroquine.

Reference:
https://www.medicines.org.uk/emc/product/5494/smpc

7.   The Paludrine/Avloclor travel pack contains enough for an adult for a four-week holiday:

Answer: False

Rationale: It contains enough for seven weeks. One week before, a two-week holiday, and four weeks after.

8.   Insect repellents containing DEET 50% are recommended:

Answer: True

9.   The strength of Viagra Connect is 100 mg:

Answer: False

Rationale: It is 50 mg.

Reference:
https://www.medicines.org.uk/emc/product/8725

10.   Sumatriptan is licensed for ages 18-60:

Answer: False

Rationale: It is 18-65.

Reference:
https://www.medicines.org.uk/emc/product/3463

11.   Chloramphenicol eye ointment should be kept in the fridge:

Answer: False

Rationale: Chloramphenicol eye drops should be kept in the fridge.

Reference:
https://www.medicines.org.uk/emc/product/7299

12.   The minimum age for orlistat is 16 years:

Answer: False

Rationale: It is 18

Reference:
https://www.medicines.org.uk/emc/product/6533/smpc

13.   The maximum age for orlistat is 60:

Answer: False

Rationale: There is no maximum age. Only certain drugs have them.

14.   Orlistat 120 mg capsules are available to buy:

Answer: False

Rationale: 60 mg capsules are available to buy.

15.   Esomeprazole, omeprazole, and pantoprazole are all P meds:

Answer: False

Rationale: Esomeprazole is GSL and is available as Nexium Control and omeprazole is also GSL and available as Pyrocalm Control. Pantoprazole is available as a P med called Pantoloc Control.

Reference:
https://www.medicines.org.uk/emc/product/3660/smpc
https://www.medicines.org.uk/emc/product/9154/smpc#gref
https://www.medicines.org.uk/emc/product/493

16.   Chlorphenamine is no longer recommended for cough and cold in under 6s:

Answer: True

Reference: https://www.gov.uk/drug-safety-update/over-the-counter-cough-and-cold-medicines-for-children

17.   Simple Linctus is licensed from 6 years:

Answer: False

Rationale: It is licensed from 12 years.

Reference:
https://www.medicines.org.uk/emc/product/4925/smpc

18.   Simple Paediatric Linctus is licensed from birth:

Answer: False

Rationale: It is licensed from 1 year.

Reference:
https://www.medicines.org.uk/emc/product/4935

19. Oral decongestants should not be used for more than 7 days:
Answer: False
Rationale: This applies to nasal decongestants as it can cause rebound congestion.

20. Ipratropium is available OTC in a combination nasal spray with xylometazoline:
Answer: True
Rationale: It is marketed as Otrivine Extra Dual Relief Nasal Spray.
Reference:
https://www.medicines.org.uk/emc/product/10022

21. Hydrocortisone 2.5 mg Muco-Adhesive Buccal Tablets are available OTC:
Answer: True
Reference:
https://www.medicines.org.uk/emc/product/5037/smpc

22. Decongestants can cause drowsiness:
Answer: False

23. Sodium chloride nasal drops are safe to use from birth:
Answer: True

24. Coloured sputum is very common and indicates the need for antibiotics:
Answer: False

25.   A patient with a cough lasting over a week should be referred to their GP:

Answer: False

Rationale: It is three weeks.

26.   Pink frothy sputum can be seen in heart failure:

Answer: True

27.   The MHRA advises that Codeine Linctus should not be used in children under 12:

Answer: False

Rationale: It is children under 18.

Reference:
https://assets.publishing.service.gov.uk/government/upl oads/system/uploads/attachment_data/file/852402/Oral_ liquid_cough_medicines_containing_codeine_should_no t_be_used_in_those_aged_less_than_18_years.pdf

28.   Dextromethorphan is more potent than codeine and pholcodine:

Answer: False

Rationale: It is less potent.

29.   The active ingredient in Simple Linctus is glycerol:

Answer: False

Rationale: It is citric acid monohydrate.

30.   Diphenhydramine is an ingredient in cough mixtures:
Answer: True
Rationale: It is contained in Benylin Chesty Cough Original.
Reference:
https://www.medicines.org.uk/emc/product/1476

31.   Guaifenesin is a cough suppressant:
Answer: False
Rationale: It is an expectorant.

32.   90% of sore throats are due to a bacterial infection:
Answer: False
Rationale: They are due to viral infections.

33.   Patients who take carbimazole and present with a sore throat should be referred immediately:
Answer: True
Reference:
https://bnf.nice.org.uk/drug/carbimazole.html

34.   Infectious mononucleosis is common in the elderly:
Answer: False
Rationale: It is common in 15-25-year-olds and is also known as the Glandular fever/kissing disease.
Reference: https://patient.info/ears-nose-throat-mouth/sore-throat-2/glandular-fever-infectious-mononucleosis

35.   Presence of cough is part of the CENTOR criteria:

Answer: False

Rationale: Absence of cough

Reference: https://cks.nice.org.uk/topics/sore-throat-acute/diagnosis/diagnosing-the-cause/

36.   Flurbiprofen lozenges are licensed from 12 years:

Answer: True

Reference: https://www.medicines.org.uk/emc/product/6514

37.   Beechams All-in-One Oral solution contains 19% v/v alcohol:

Answer: True

Rationale: A 20 mL dose is equal to 76 mL beer and this is a GSL product!

Reference: https://www.medicines.org.uk/emc/product/3913/smpc

38.   Acrivastine is a sedating antihistamine:

Answer: False

39.   Cetirizine can be used in children over 2:

Answer: True

Reference: https://www.medicines.org.uk/emc/product/4568

40.	Loratadine can be used in children under 2:
Answer: False
Reference:
https://www.medicines.org.uk/emc/product/8807/smpc

41.	Acrivastine can be used in children over 12:
Answer: True
Reference:
https://www.medicines.org.uk/emc/product/3388/smpc

42.	Chlorphenamine can be used from 1 year in children suffering from an allergy:
Answer: True
Reference:
https://www.medicines.org.uk/emc/product/3928/smpc

43.	There are five steroid nasal sprays available OTC:
Answer: True

44.	Beclometasone, budesonide, fluticasone, hydrocortisone and mometasone nasal sprays are available OTC:
Answer: False
Rationale: Triamcinolone not hydrocortisone.
Reference:
https://www.medicines.org.uk/emc/product/26
https://www.benadryl.co.uk/products/prevention/benacort-nasal-spray
https://www.medicines.org.uk/emc/product/4502/smpc
https://www.medicines.org.uk/emc/product/6501

https://www.claritynallergy.co.uk/products/clarinaze/

45.   OTC steroid nasal sprays are licensed from 16 years:
Answer: False
Rationale: 18 years

46.   Azelastine nasal spray is available OTC:
Answer: False
Rationale: It is a POM.

47.   You can sell a pack of 24 x 30 mg pseudoephedrine tablets:
Answer: True
Reference: https://www.gov.uk/drug-safety-update/pseudoephedrine-and-ephedrine-regular-review-of-minimising-risk-of-misuse-in-the-uk

48.   Otrivine Extra Dual Relief Nasal Spray is licensed from 12 years:
Answer: False
Rationale: 18 years. It contains ipratropium/xylometazoline

49.   Lidocaine throat sprays are licensed from 12 years:
Answer: True
Reference:
https://www.medicines.org.uk/emc/product/4834/smpc

50.   Eye drops containing naphazoline can be used from 12 years:
Answer: True
Reference:
https://www.medicines.org.uk/emc/product/5640

51.   There are no ocular antihistamines available OTC:
Answer: False
Rationale: Antalozine/xylometazoline
Reference:
https://www.medicines.org.uk/emc/product/6294

52.   Chloramphenicol can be used OTC from 1 year:
Answer: False
Rationale: 2 years
Reference:
https://www.medicines.org.uk/emc/product/612/smpc

53. Chloramphenicol ointment should only be applied at night when used with drops:
Answer: True
Reference:
https://www.medicines.org.uk/emc/product/7299/smpc

54.   Chloramphenicol eye drops can be used for up to 7 days:
Answer: False
5 days

55.   Sodium cromoglicate eye drops should only be used once daily:
Answer: False
Rationale: Four times
Reference:
https://www.medicines.org.uk/emc/product/1944

56.   There is a risk of severe and fatal burns with steroid creams:
Answer: False
Rationale: Paraffin based emollients
Reference: https://www.gov.uk/drug-safety-update/emollients-new-information-about-risk-of-severe-and-fatal-burns-with-paraffin-containing-and-paraffin-free-emollients

57.   Oral lidocaine-containing products are GSL:
Answer: False
Rationale: They are now P medicines
Reference: https://www.gov.uk/drug-safety-update/oral-lidocaine-containing-products-for-infant-teething-only-to-be-available-under-the-supervision-of-a-pharmacist

58.   Some head lice products are combustible/flammable when used on hair:
Answer: True
Reference: https://www.gov.uk/drug-safety-update/head-lice-eradication-products-risk-of-serious-burns-if-treated-hair-is-exposed-to-open-flames-or-other-sources-of-ignition-eg-cigarettes

59.   Miconazole oral gel is contraindicated in patients who are taking warfarin:

Answer: True

Reference: https://www.gov.uk/drug-safety-update/miconazole-daktarin-over-the-counter-oral-gel-contraindicated-in-patients-taking-warfarin

60.   Overdose of loperamide can lead to serious hepatic events:

Answer: False

Rationale: Cardiac

Reference: https://www.gov.uk/drug-safety-update/loperamide-imodium-reports-of-serious-cardiac-adverse-reactions-with-high-doses-of-loperamide-associated-with-abuse-or-misuse

61.   Co-codamol 8/500 mg tablets can be used by a 12-year-old if they do not have breathing problems:

Answer: True

Reference: https://www.gov.uk/drug-safety-update/codeine-for-cough-and-cold-restricted-use-in-children

62.   Co-codamol 8/500 mg tablets are licensed for sore throats:

Answer: False

Reference: https://www.gov.uk/drug-safety-update/over-the-counter-painkillers-containing-codeine-or-dihydrocodeine

63.   The maximum pack size for paracetamol/dihydrocodeine tablets is 24:
Answer: False
Rationale: 32
Reference: https://www.medicines.org.uk/emc/product/1309

64.   Paramol tablets contain paracetamol 500 mg and dihydrocodeine 10 mg:
Answer: False
Rationale: 7.46 mg

65.   There is no treatment available for mild Otitis Externa:
Answer: False
Rationale: EarCalm Spray (2% acetic acid spray is available and recommended for 7 days
Reference: https://www.medicines.org.uk/emc/product/9013

66.   Migraine with aura is classed as a primary headache according to the International Headache Society:
Answer: True
Reference: Rutter, Paul. Community Pharmacy, Symptoms, Diagnosis and Treatment 2020

67.   Migraines are more common in men than women:
Answer: False
Reference: https://www.nhs.uk/conditions/migraine/

68.   Cluster headaches are more common in men than women:

Answer: True

https://www.nhs.uk/conditions/cluster-headaches/

69.   The most common type of headache seen in community pharmacy is tension-type headache:

Answer: True

Reference: Rutter, Paul. Community Pharmacy, Symptoms, Diagnosis and Treatment 2020

70.   Headache with aura is more common than without aura:

Answer: False

Reference: https://www.nhs.uk/conditions/migraine/

71.   Subarachnoid haemorrhages are more common in black people compared to other ethnic groups.

Answer: True

Reference:
https://www.nhs.uk/conditions/subarachnoid-haemorrhage/

72.   Migraleve Pink tablets contain 8/500 co-codamol:

Answer: False

Rationale: They also contain buclizine 6.25 mg

Reference:
https://www.medicines.org.uk/emc/product/1188

73.   Buccastem M should only be used for a maximum of three days:
Answer: False
Rationale: Two
Reference:
https://www.medicines.org.uk/emc/product/478

74.   Buccastem M should be swallowed whole with a full glass of water:
Answer: False
Rationale: It should be placed high along the top gum under the upper lip.

75.   Sumatriptan 100 mg is OTC:
Answer: False
Rationale: 50 mg
Reference:
https://www.medicines.org.uk/emc/product/3463/smpc

76.   The maximum number of sumatriptan tablets that can be taken each day is two:
Answer: True

77.   Diphenhydramine and promethazine tablets can be sold to patients aged 18 and over for insomnia:
Answer: False
Rationale: It is 16.
Reference:
https://www.medicines.org.uk/emc/product/340/smpc
https://www.medicines.org.uk/emc/product/9010

78.   Alkalinizing agents for cystitis should be taken for three days:
Answer: False
Rationale: It is two.
Reference:
https://www.canesten.co.uk/en/female/products/canesoasis-cystitis-relief/

79.   Thrush has a thin white discharge and a strong fishy odour:
Answer: False
Rationale: Bacterial vaginosis
Reference: https://www.nhs.uk/conditions/bacterial-vaginosis/

80.   Clotrimazole pessaries should be used in the morning:
Answer: False
Rationale: Evening
Reference:
https://www.medicines.org.uk/emc/product/11464/smpc

81.   Fluconazole oral capsules are licensed for use in women only:
Answer: False
Reference:
https://www.medicines.org.uk/emc/product/40

82.   Vaginal thrush products can only be sold to those aged 16-60:
Answer: True
Reference: https://www.nhs.uk/conditions/thrush-in-men-and-women/

83.   **Treatment with orlistat may potentially impair the absorption of water-soluble vitamins.**
Answer: False
Rationale: Fat soluble vitamins
Reference:
https://www.medicines.org.uk/emc/product/6533

84.   No more than three orlistat capsules should be taken in a 24-hour period:
Answer: True

85.   Buscopan Cramps are contraindicated in patients with myasthenia gravis:
Answer: True
Reference:
https://www.medicines.org.uk/emc/product/891

86.   The maximum daily dose of tranexamic acid is 3 g:
Answer: False
Rationale: 4 g
Reference:
https://www.medicines.org.uk/emc/product/1768/smpc

87.   Tranexamic acid should be used for a maximum of 3 days:
Answer: False
4 days

88.   The initial dosage of tranexamic acid tablets is one tablet three times daily:
Answer: False
Rationale: Two tablets three times daily

89.   Painless mouth ulcers must be referred:
Answer: True
Rationale: It could be a sign of something more serious.
Reference: https://patient.info/doctor/oral-ulceration

90.   Minor aphthous ulcers normally resolve in 2-3 days:
Answer: False
Rationale: 7-14 days
Reference: https://www.nhs.uk/conditions/mouth-ulcers/

91.   Choline salicylate gel can be used from 6 years:
Answer: False
Rationale: 16 years
Reference:
https://www.medicines.org.uk/emc/product/624/smpc

92.   Hydrocortisone mucoadhesive buccal tablets can be used for up to 5 days:

Answer: True

Reference:
https://www.medicines.org.uk/emc/product/5037/smpc

93.   Chlorhexidine mouthwash can cause tooth discolouration:

Answer: True

Reference:
https://www.medicines.org.uk/emc/product/529/smpc

94.   Daktarin Oral Gel can be used from 1 year:

Answer: False

Rationale: 4 months

Reference:
https://www.medicines.org.uk/emc/product/6597

95.   When using Daktarin Sugar Free 2% Oral Gel, the treatment should be continued for at least a week after the symptoms have disappeared:

Answer: True

96.   Magnesium antacids can cause constipation:

Answer: False

Rationale: Diarrhoea

97.   Aluminium antacids can cause constipation:

Answer: True

98.   Ranitidine can be used from 12 years:
Answer: False
Rationale: 16
Reference:
https://www.medicines.org.uk/emc/product/55

99.   Proton Pump Inhibitors can be used from 16 years:
Answer: False
Rationale: 18 years
Reference:
https://www.medicines.org.uk/emc/product/3660/smpc

100.   Oral rehydration salts should be made with 200 mL water:
Answer: True
Reference:
https://www.medicines.org.uk/emc/product/2775/smpc

101.   The maximum daily dose of loperamide is 16 mg daily:
Answer: False
Rationale: It is 12 mg OTC
Reference:
https://www.medicines.org.uk/emc/product/522/smpc

102.   Loperamide can be used from 6 years:
Answer: False
Rationale: 12

103.   Pepto-Bismol can cause black stools:
Answer: True
Reference: https://www.nhs.uk/medicines/pepto-bismol/

104.   Kaolin and morphine is the first line treatment for diarrhoea:
Answer: False
Rationale: Subject to abuse

105.   There are three classes of OTC laxatives:
Answer: False
Rationale: Four
Reference: https://www.nhs.uk/conditions/laxatives/

106.   Lactulose is an osmotic laxative:
Answer: True

107.   Ispaghula husk is a stimulant laxative:
Answer: False
Rationale: Bulk-forming

108.   Bulk-forming laxatives can take up to 72 hours to start working:
Answer: True

109.   Stimulant laxatives take between 6-12 hours to work:
Answer: True

110. Glycerol suppositories work within seconds:
Answer: False
Rationale: 15-30 mins

111. The standard dose of senna for adults is 3 tablets at night:
Answer: False
Rationale: 2

112. Ispaghula husk should not be taken at night:
Answer: True
Reference:
https://www.medicines.org.uk/emc/product/1447/smpc

113. Lactulose is not safe in pregnancy:
Answer: False
Reference:
https://www.medicines.org.uk/emc/product/5525/smpc

114. Docusate sodium is an osmotic laxative:
Answer: False
Rationale: Stool softener
Reference:
https://www.medicines.org.uk/emc/product/212/smpc#P
RODUCTINFO

115.   Hyoscine butylbromide can be used from 6 years:

Answer: True

Rationale: Although this relates to Buscopan Cramps which is a P med and not to Buscopan IBS Relief which is GSL

Reference: https://www.medicines.org.uk/emc/product/891

116.   Alverine and mebeverine can both be used in those over 12:

Answer: False

Rationale: Mebeverine is 18

Reference: https://www.medicines.org.uk/emc/product/1898/smpc

117.   Peru balsam is a protectant used in haemorrhoid preparations:

Answer: False

Rationale: Astringent

Reference: Rutter, Paul. Community Pharmacy, Symptoms, Diagnosis and Treatment 2020

118.   Budesonide is available as a GSL nasal spray.

Answer: True

Reference: https://www.gov.uk/government/publications/public-assessment-report-of-the-reclassification-of-benacort-hayfever-relief-for-adults-64-micrograms-nasal-spray-from-pom-to-gsl

119.   Haemorrhoid products containing hydrocortisone should only be used for a maximum of 7 days:
Answer: True
Reference:
https://cks.nice.org.uk/topics/haemorrhoids/prescribing-information/topical-haemorrhoidal-preparations/

120.   The most common form of psoriasis is scalp psoriasis:
Answer: False
Rationale: Plaque
Reference: https://www.psoriasis-association.org.uk/psoriasis-and-treatments/types-of-psoriasis

121.   Erythema means localised damage to the skin due to scratching:
Answer: False
Rationale: Redness due to dilated blood vessels that blanch when pressed
Reference: Rutter, Paul. Community Pharmacy, Symptoms, Diagnosis and Treatment 2020

122. There are four non-sedating antihistamines available OTC.
Answer: True
Acrivastine, cetirizine, fexofenadine and loratadine
https://www.gov.uk/government/publications/public-assessment-report-of-the-reclassification-of-allevia-120mg-tablets/par-reclassification-of-allevia-120mg-tablets-from-prescription-only-medicine-pom-to-general-sales-list-gsl

123. Ketoconazole shampoo should be used twice a week initially for the treatment of dandruff:
Answer: True
Reference:
https://www.medicines.org.uk/emc/files/pil.8269.pdf

124. Terbinafine is an imidazole:
Answer: False
Rationale: It is an Allylamine
Reference:
https://www.medicines.org.uk/emc/product/6325

125. Daktacort Hydrocortisone cream is licensed from 10 years:
Answer: True
Reference:
https://www.medicines.org.uk/emc/product/1557

126.   There are 6 classes of antifungal medicines available:

Answer: True

Rationale: Allylamines, imidazole's, benzoic acid, griseofulvin, undecanoates and tolnaftate

Reference: Rutter, Paul. Community Pharmacy, Symptoms, Diagnosis and Treatment 2020

127.   Amorolfine is used daily for distal lateral subungal onychomycosis:

Answer: False

Rationale: It is used weekly

Reference:
https://www.medicines.org.uk/emc/product/7414

128.   Amorolfine is licensed from 18 years:

Answer: True

129.   Toenails take approximately 6 months to regrow:

Answer: False

Rationale: 9-12 months

Reference: Rutter, Paul. Community Pharmacy, Symptoms, Diagnosis and Treatment 2020, Paul. Community Pharmacy, Symptoms, Diagnosis and Treatment 2020

130.   Each pack of amorolfine provides one month's treatment:

Answer: False

Rationale: It provides 3 months treatment.

131. Minoxidil should be applied to the scalp three times daily:

Answer: False

Rationale: It should be applied twice daily

Reference:
https://www.medicines.org.uk/emc/product/5765/smpc

132. Minoxidil 5% is only licensed for men:

Answer: True

Rationale: 2% licensed for women.

Reference:
https://www.medicines.org.uk/emc/product/102/smpc

133. Minoxidil is licensed from 18 years to 65 years:

Answer: True

134. Warts and verrucae are caused by the varicella zoster virus:

Answer: False

Rationale: They are caused by the Human Papilloma virus

Reference: https://www.nhsinform.scot/illnesses-and-conditions/skin-hair-and-nails/warts-and-verrucas

135. Salicylic acid products for warts and verrucae should be used once daily:

Answer: True

Reference:
https://www.medicines.org.uk/emc/product/296/smpc

136.   Glutaraldehyde should be used once daily:

Answer: False

Rationale: Twice daily

Reference:
https://www.medicines.org.uk/emc/product/3758

137.   Permethrin cream should be used from the neck down for scabies in all adults:

Answer: False

Rationale: Manufacturer says neck down but BNF says to ignore this and apply all over the head but avoiding the eyes. The manufacturer also states that in the elderly, the face, ears and scalp should also be treated.

138.   Permethrin cream is licensed for use from 2 years:

Answer: False

Rationale: 2 months

Reference:
https://www.medicines.org.uk/emc/product/1715

139.   Cold sores are caused by the herpes simplex virus:

Answer: True

140.   Aciclovir should be used four times daily for five days:

Answer: False

Five times daily

Reference:
https://www.medicines.org.uk/emc/product/27/smpc

141.   Penciclovir cream is used eight times daily:
Answer: True
Reference:
https://www.medicines.org.uk/emc/product/6338

142.   Hydrocortisone cream can only be used from 10 years:
Answer: True
Reference:
https://www.medicines.org.uk/emc/product/5651

143.   A maximum of 30 g hydrocortisone cream can be sold at one time:
Answer: False
Rationale: 15 g

144.   Hydrocortisone cream is available to buy for use on the ears:
Answer: True
Rationale: Ears are not part of the face.

145.   Clobetasol cream is available to buy:
Answer: False
Clobetasone
Reference:
https://www.medicines.org.uk/emc/product/3929

146.   Clobetasone cream can be used from 10 years
Answer: False
Rationale: 12 years

147.   There is a combination aspirin and paracetamol product available:
Answer: True
Rationale: Anadin Extra
Reference:
https://www.medicines.org.uk/emc/product/11893/smpc

148.   Solpadeine Plus and Solpadeine Max contain the same amount of codeine:
Answer: False
Rationale: Solpadeine Plus contains 8 mg and Max 12.8 mg
Reference:
https://www.medicines.org.uk/emc/product/6488
https://www.medicines.org.uk/emc/product/3923/smpc

149.   Ibuprofen suspension is available in 100 mg/5 mL and 200 mg/5 mL
Answer: True
Rationale:

150.   Dimeticone 4% lotion can be used from 1 year:
Answer: False
Rationale: 6 months
Reference:
https://www.medicines.org.uk/emc/product/4901/smpc

151.   Everyone in the house should be treated at the same time for head lice:

Answer: False

Rationale: Just the affected individual

152.   Head lice treatments should be re-applied after 7 days:

Answer: True

Reference: Rutter, Paul. Community Pharmacy, Symptoms, Diagnosis and Treatment 2020

153.   Head lice are only associated with dirty hair:

Answer: False

Reference: https://www.chemistanddruggist.co.uk/content/how-to-recognise-and-treat-headlice

154.   Children with head lice should be kept off school:

Answer: False

155.   Isopropyl myristate can be used from two years:

Answer: True

Rationale: Full Marks Solution Spray

https://patient.info/childrens-health/head-lice-and-nits/treating-and-preventing-head-lice-and-nits

156.   Isopropyl myristate should be left on for 30 minutes:

Answer: False

Rationale: 5-10 mins

157.   Everyone in the house should be treated at the same time for threadworm:
Answer: True
Reference:
https://www.medicines.org.uk/emc/product/1317/smpc

158.   Mebendazole can be used from 6 months:
Answer: False
Rationale: 2 years

159.   The mebendazole dose for adults and children is the same:
Answer: True
Rationale: 100 mg

160.   Infacol is safe to use from birth for colic:
Answer: True
Simeticone
Reference: https://www.infacol.co.uk/

161.   Gripe water is safe to use from birth:
Answer: False
Rationale: 1 month
Reference:
https://www.medicines.org.uk/emc/product/3611

162.   Colief contains simeticone:
Answer: False
Rationale: lactase
Reference: https://colief.co.uk/

163. Emollients should be used sparingly:
Answer: False
Reference: https://www.nhs.uk/conditions/emollients/

164. A three-year-old should take 7.5 mL of paracetamol 120 mg/5 mL oral suspension:
Answer: True
Reference:
https://www.medicines.org.uk/emc/product/5908

165. A four-year-old should take 7.5 mL of ibuprofen 100 mg/5 mL suspension:
Answer: True
Reference:
https://www.medicines.org.uk/emc/product/8139

166. Chickenpox is caused by the herpes zoster virus:
Answer: False
Rationale: Varicella zoster
Reference: https://patient.info/doctor/chickenpox-pro

167. Molluscum contagiosum is a bacterial infection:
Answer: False
Rationale: Pox virus
Reference: https://patient.info/childrens-health/viral-skin-infections-leaflet/molluscum-contagiosum

168.   First line treatment for **non-bullous** impetigo is Crystacide cream:
Answer: True
Rationale: NICE
Reference:
https://www.nice.org.uk/guidance/ng153/resources/visual-summary-pdf-7084853533

169.   Glandular fever is caused by the Epstein-Barr virus:
Answer: True
Reference: https://patient.info/ears-nose-throat-mouth/sore-throat-2/glandular-fever-infectious-mononucleosis

170.   Scarlet fever is a viral infection:
Answer: False
Rationale: Bacterial
Reference: https://patient.info/skin-conditions/viral-rashes/scarlet-fever

171.   Roseola infantum is a viral infection:
Answer: True
Rationale: human herpesvirus 6
Reference: https://patient.info/skin-conditions/viral-rashes/roseola

172.   Roseola infantum is also called sixth disease:
Answer: True

173.   A blanching rash can occur with meningitis:
Answer: False
Rationale: Non-blanching
Reference: https://cks.nice.org.uk/topics/meningitis-bacterial-meningitis-meningococcal-disease/diagnosis/assessing-the-rash/

174.   German measles is also known as rubella:
Answer: True
Reference: https://patient.info/skin-conditions/viral-rashes/rubella-german-measles

175.   Mumps is much more unpleasant if contracted as a child:
Answer: False
Rationale: Adult
Reference: https://patient.info/travel-and-vaccinations/mumps-leaflet

176.   Measles has an incubation period of one to two days:
Answer: False
Rationale: One to two weeks
Reference: https://patient.info/skin-conditions/viral-rashes/measles

177.   Koplik's spots occur in Measles:
Answer: True

178.   Scarlet fever is also called slapped cheek disease:
Answer: False
Rationale: Erythema infectiosum
Reference: https://patient.info/childrens-health/slapped-cheek-disease-leaflet

179.   Erythema infectiosum is also known as fifth disease:
Answer: True

180.   Glandular fever is a notifiable disease:
Answer: False
Rationale: Scarlet fever

181.   Glandular fever is also called the kissing disease:
Answer: True

182.   Mumps is the most contagious of the childhood diseases:
Answer: False
Rationale: Least
Reference: Rutter, Paul. Community Pharmacy, Symptoms, Diagnosis and Treatment 2020

183.   Joy-Rides can be used from 4 years:
Answer: False
Rationale: 3 years
Reference:
https://www.medicines.org.uk/emc/product/9016

184.   Kwells Kids can be used from 5 years:
Answer: False
Rationale: 4 years
Reference:
https://www.medicines.org.uk/emc/product/252/smpc

185.   Hyoscine does not cross the blood-barrier:
Answer: False

186.   A hyoscine patch is available for motion
sickness:
Answer: True
Rationale: Scopoderm
Reference:
https://www.medicines.org.uk/emc/product/3276

187.   Kwells can be used from 10 years:
Answer: True
Reference:
https://www.medicines.org.uk/emc/product/250/smpc

188.   EllaOne contains levonorgestrel:
Answer: False
Rationale: Ulipristal

189.   EllaOne can be used in any female of
childbearing age:
Answer: True

190.   Ellaone can be used for up to 120 hours post unprotected sexual intercourse:
Answer: True

191.   Ulipristal does not pass into breast milk:
Answer: False

192.   Levonorgestrel can be used up to 72 hours post unprotected sexual intercourse:
Answer: True

193.   If a patient vomits within four hours of taking levonorgestrel or ulipristal, a further supply would be needed:
Answer: False
Rationale: 3 hours
Reference: https://www.fsrh.org/standards-and-guidance/documents/ceu-clinical-guidance-emergency-contraception-march-2017/

194.   Levonorgestrel is more efficacious than ulipristal:
Answer: False

195.   A maximum of two nicotine inhalation cartridges can be used in 24 hours:
Answer: False
Rationale: Six

196.   The maximum daily limit of nicotine nasal spray is 64 sprays:
Answer: True

197.   Nicotine patches should be changed every 72 hours:
Answer: False
Rationale: 24 hours

198.   Crotamiton can be used from three years:
Answer: True

199.   Large packs of stimulant laxatives are available GSL:
Answer: False
Rationale: https://www.gov.uk/drug-safety-update/stimulant-laxatives-bisacodyl-senna-and-sennosides-sodium-picosulfate-available-over-the-counter-new-measures-to-support-safe-use

200.   Children under 18 years must see a doctor if they require stimulant laxatives.
False
Rationale: Products for children aged 12 to 17 years can be supplied under the supervision of a pharmacist.

Printed in Great Britain
by Amazon

21968108R00043